THE BEST KEPT SECRET

by

DR. ANDREA AUERBACH

The Best Kept Secret

by Dr. Andrea Auerbach

Cover design and illustrations by *Brenda Brown*

ISBN-10: 1942489137;

ISBN-13: 978-1-942489-13-9

Acknowledgements

Thank you to my brother, Mitchell, who suggested that I write a chiropractic children's book.

A deep heartfelt thank you to Carol Patti for her lasting patience, valuable time, and numerous editings. Her contribution was a crucial factor in the imminent completion of this book.

Thank you to Jodie, my chiropractic assistant, for keeping me on course.

Thanks to Hilary, Tory, Jennifer, Karen, Iska, Doris, and all of the office moms and practice members who offered their invaluable suggestions and motivational support.

Special thanks to Dr. Janet Patti and Celeste Gialluca for helping me get to the finish line.

I am especially grateful for the parents who have embraced chiropractic care for their children and allowed me the privilege of caring for them.

To the children who have inspired me—thank you for making my practice so much about wellness care and for adding humor and lightness to my daily work.

This book is dedicated to Janice Garone.
She was my chiropractic assistant and a dear friend.
Janice was loved by staff and practice members alike.
Her love and laughter live on in our office and
in my heart.

The boy in this book was named after her son Justin.

THE BEST
KEPT SECRET

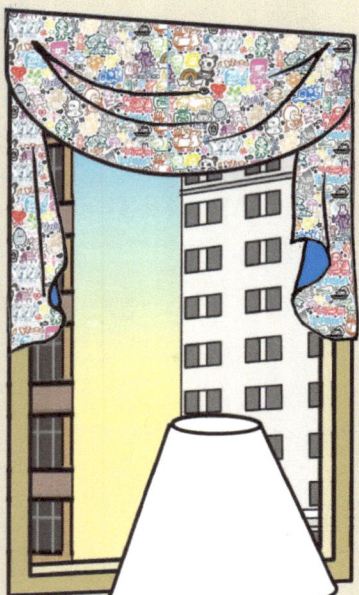

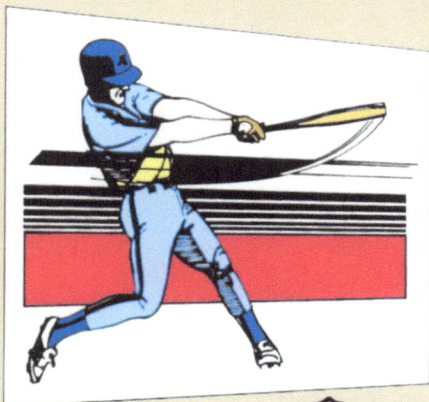

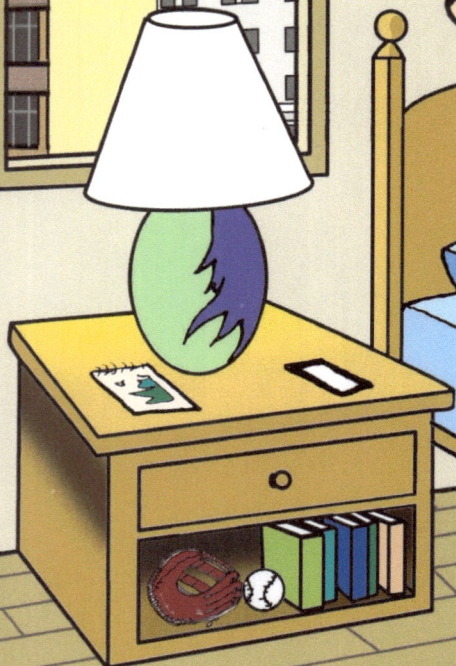

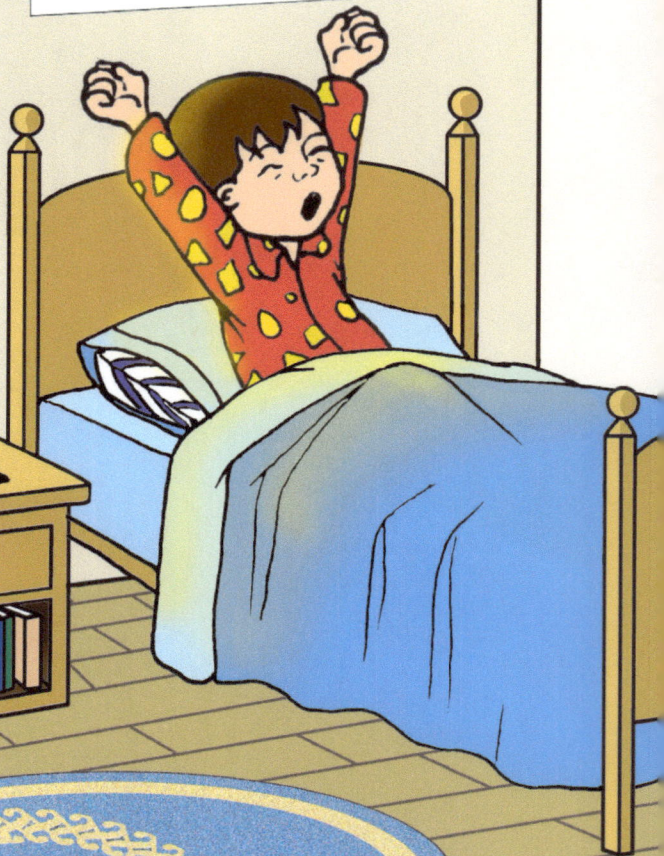

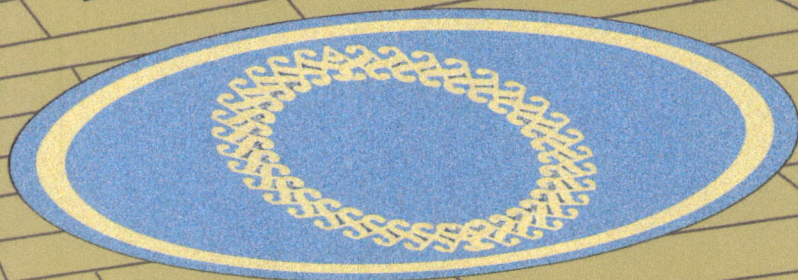

Justin woke up early,

Looking forward to his day.

He had a lot of things to do,

To see, to build, to play.

The day starts off with breakfast,

Lots of healthy foods to eat.

He sits and talks with mom and dad,

That is his favorite treat.

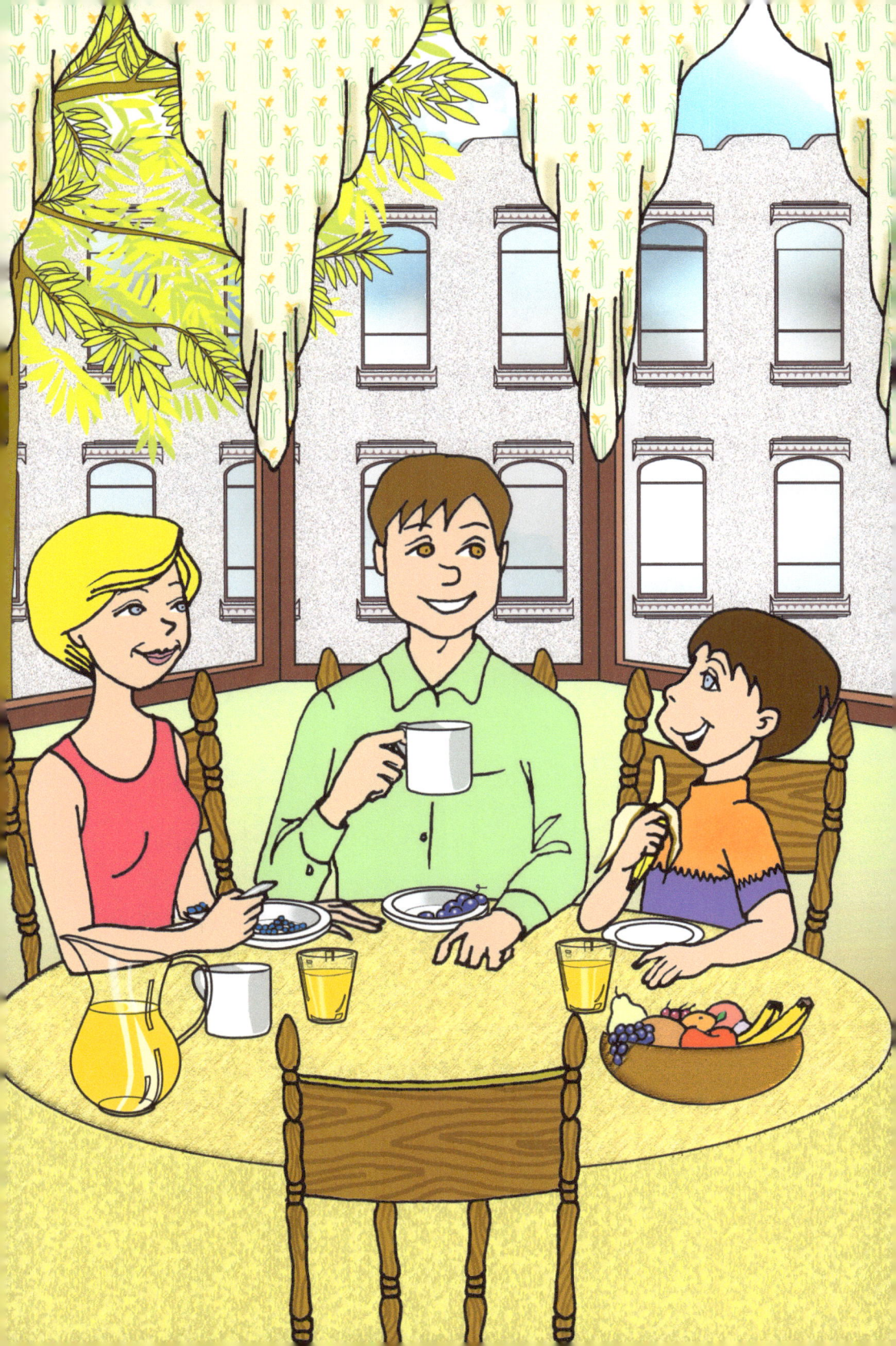

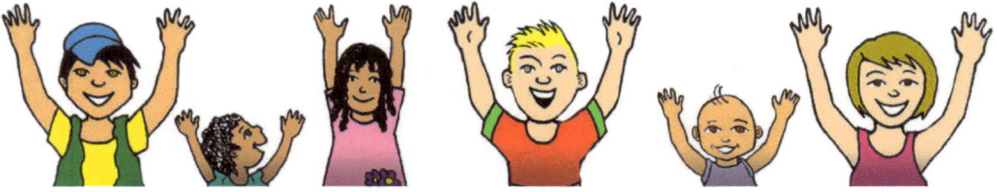

Then off to school to read and write,

There's time to laugh and play.

But seeing Doctor 'A' tonight,

Is the best part of his day.

"The other kids stay home

from school,

They're sick and cannot go.

Why don't they go to Dr. 'A',

And stay healthy, I don't know."

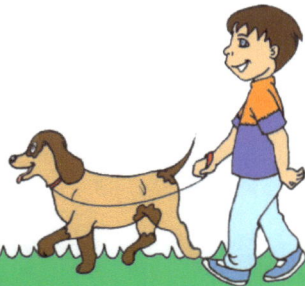

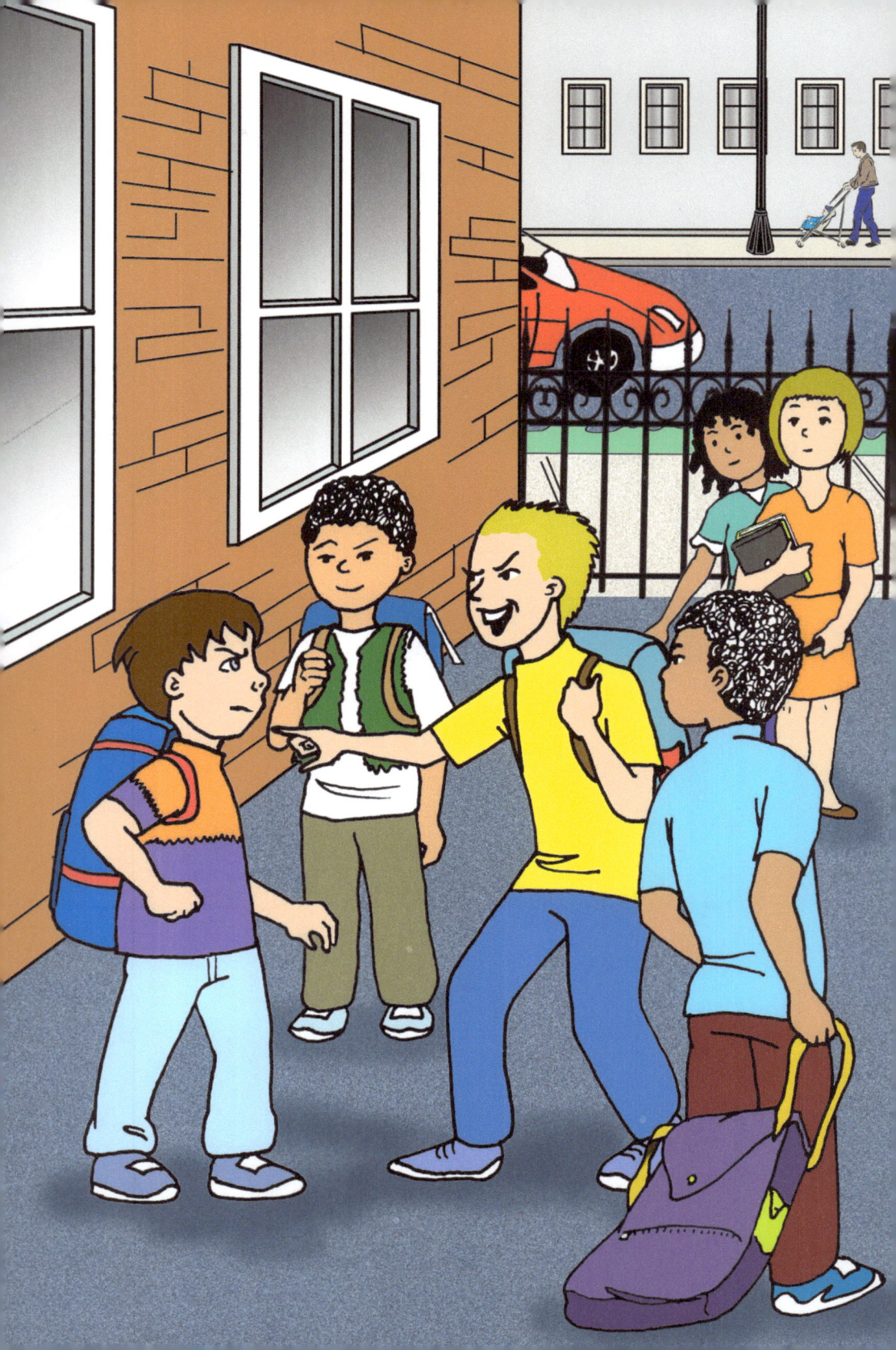

Justin went to school that day,

Feeling smart and proud.

A boy began to bully him,

His voice was very loud.

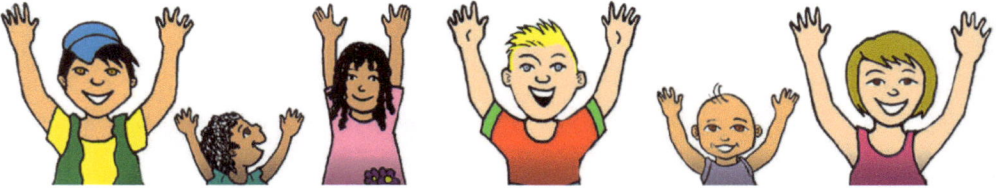

"Did you hear about Justin?"

He wanted everyone to know.

"Justin sees his doctor,

And he really LIKES to go."

"What kind of doctor could there be,

That you go to when you're well?

We're going to the teacher,

And we are going to tell."

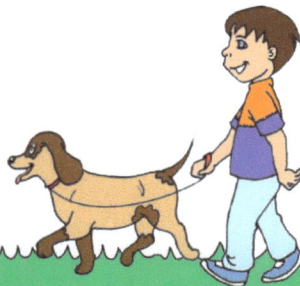

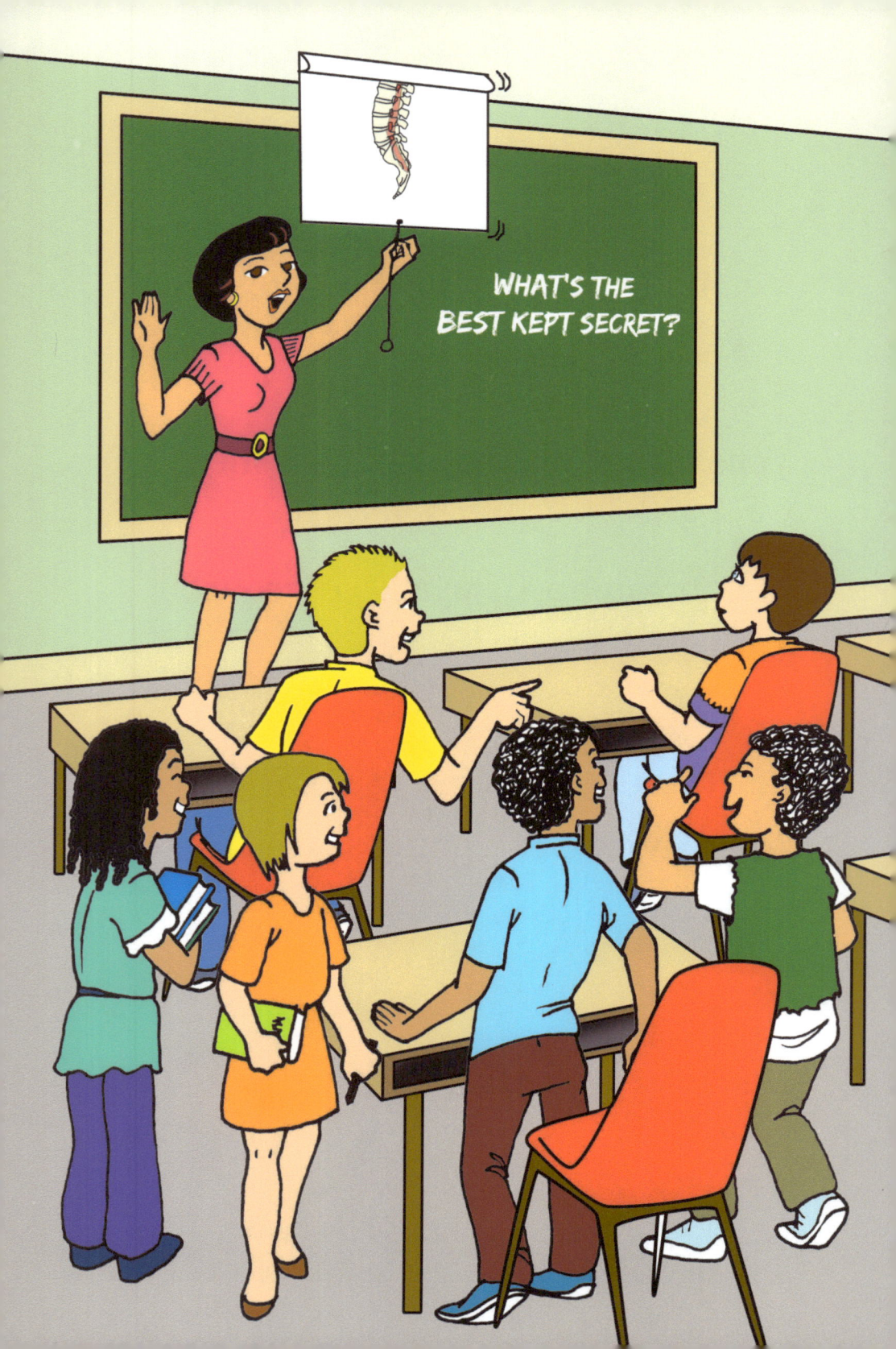

"Now, now children," the teacher said,

"The truth we always seek.

We must be fair with open mind,

So please let Justin speak."

"The brain sends signals everywhere,

My Doctor told me so.

She keeps my nervous system clear,

So messages can flow."

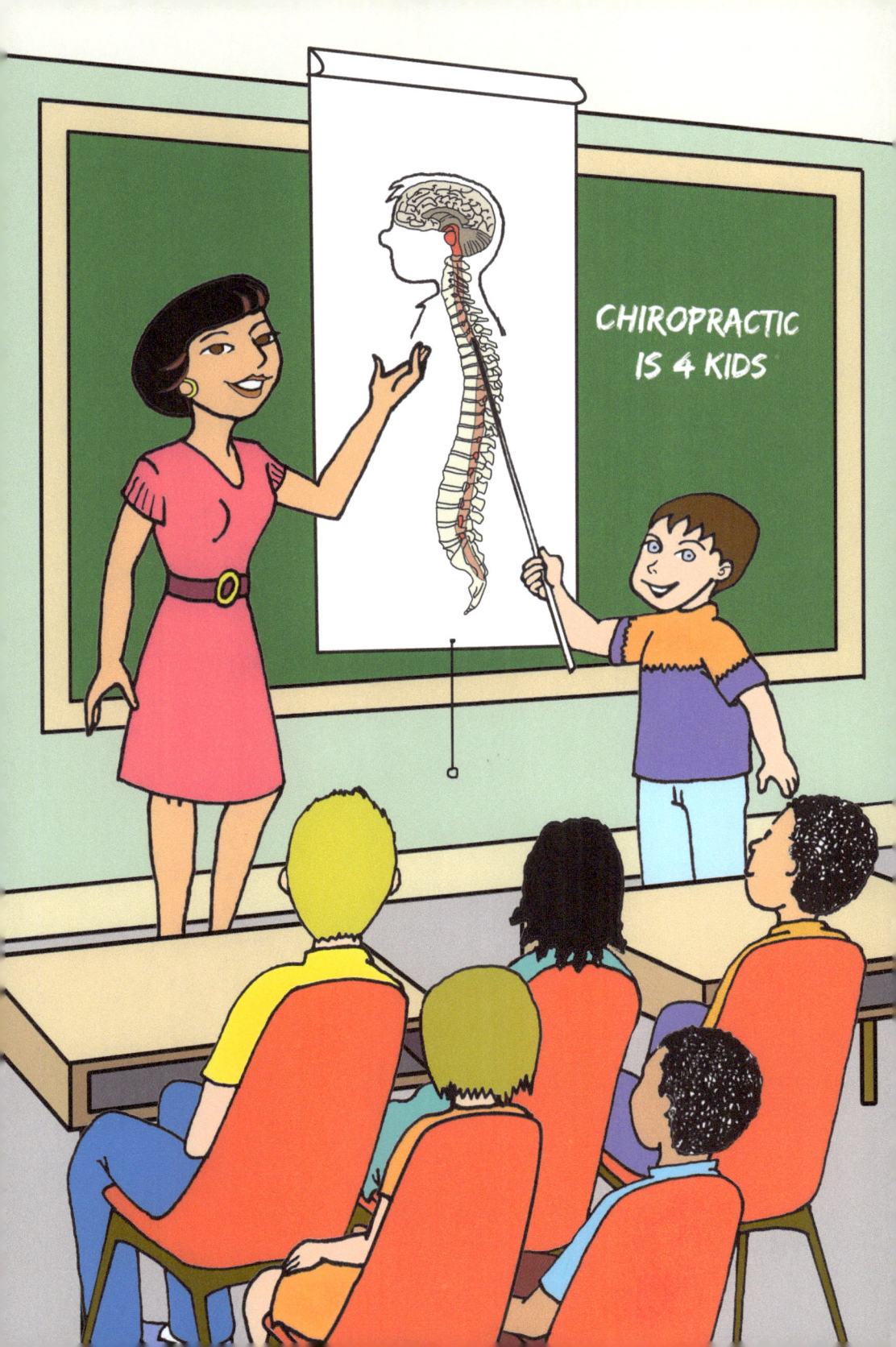

CHIROPRACTIC IS 4 KIDS

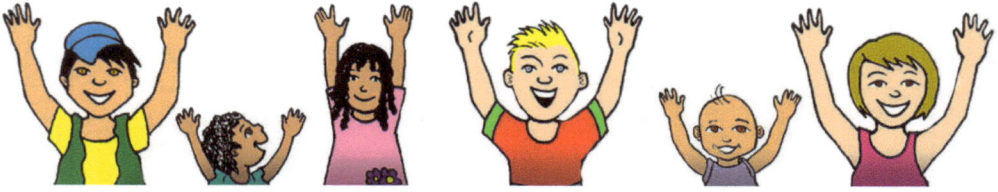

"Wellness visits are the key

To keep health in control;

Running, breathing and homework

come easy,

That's why I like to go."

The teacher called his parents,

To make sure he wasn't sick.

"They spoke about his doctor,

Have the children played a trick?"

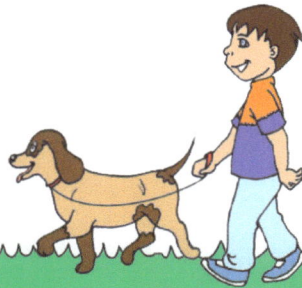

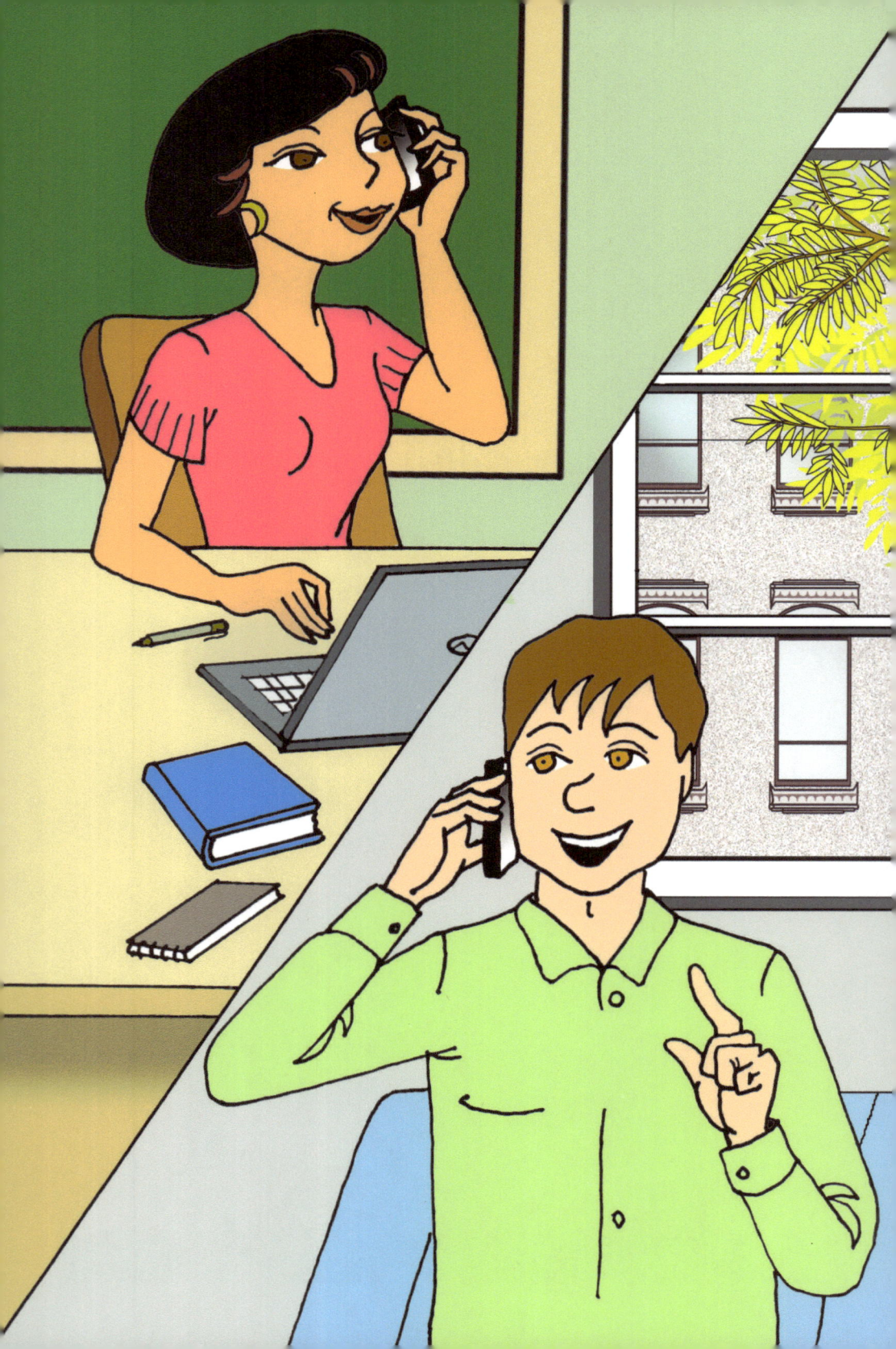

"Yes, it is true what they say,

Thank you for the call.

Since birth this doctor's kept him well,

He's hardly sick at all."

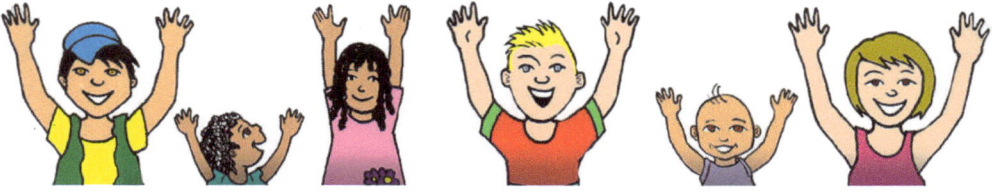

The teacher said, "Now that's a

lesson,

All of us should know.

Justin can you teach the class,

What happens when you go?"

"I climb up on the cushions,

I'm in charge there is no doubt.

I choose if I want popcorn sound,

or I can pick without."

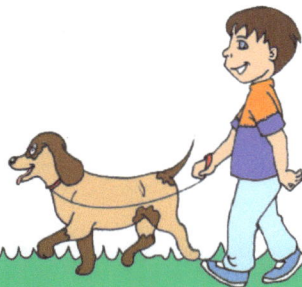

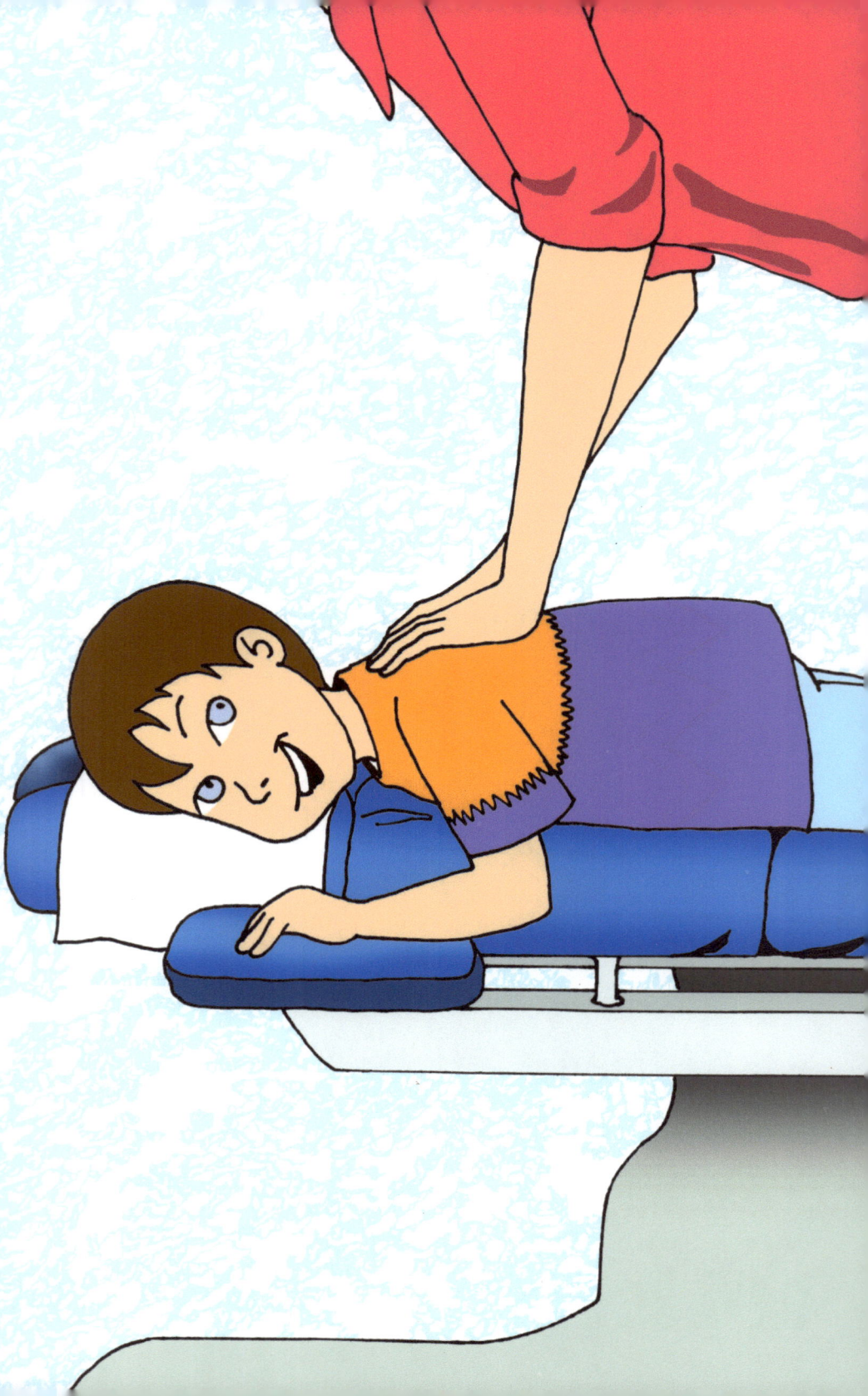

"I was a little scared at first,

She moved my head around.

She explained it wouldn't hurt,

Just make a popping sound."

"The computer and my backpack,

Are stressful on my spine.

But then I go to Dr. 'A,'

And go home feeling fine."

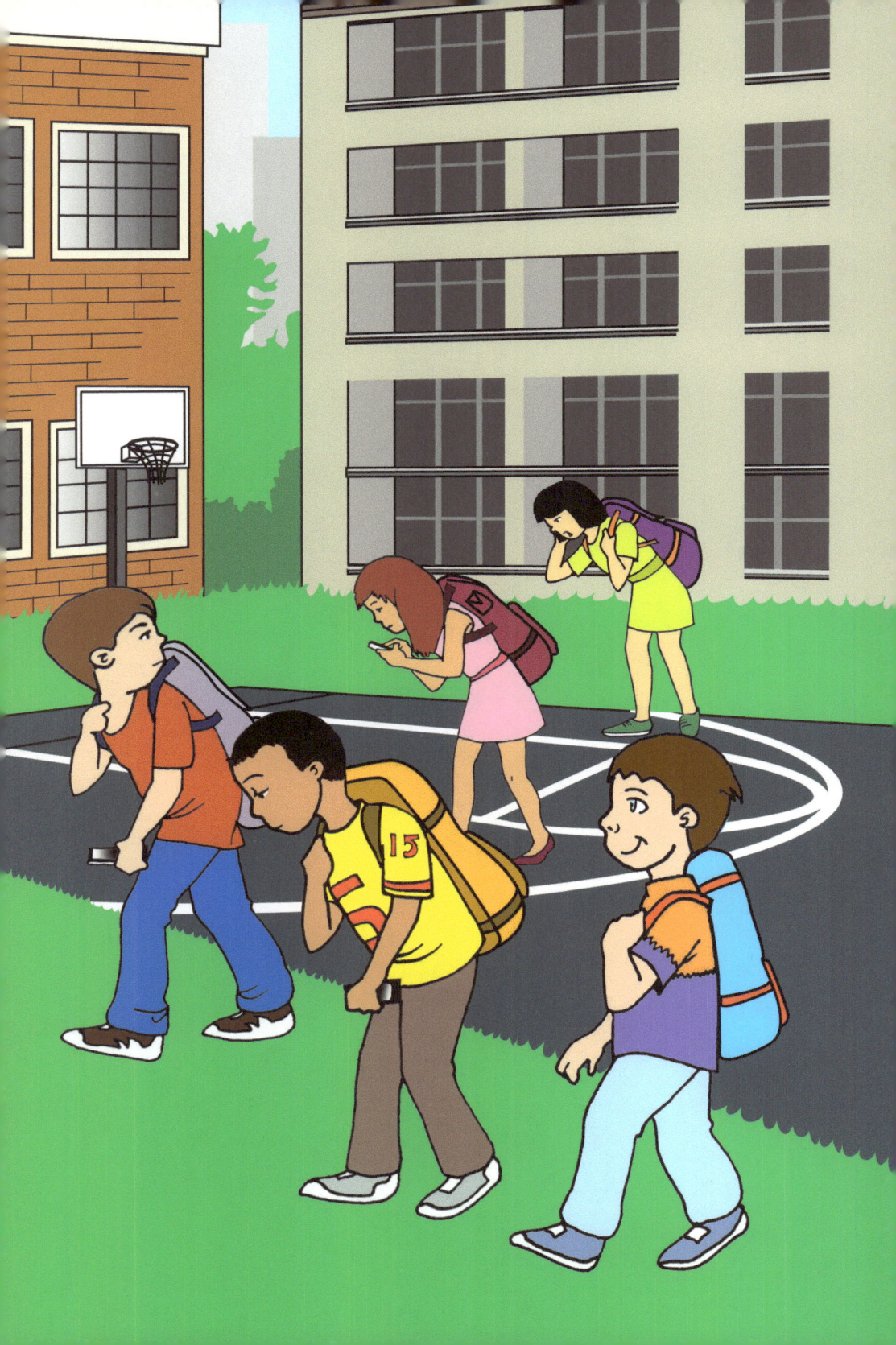

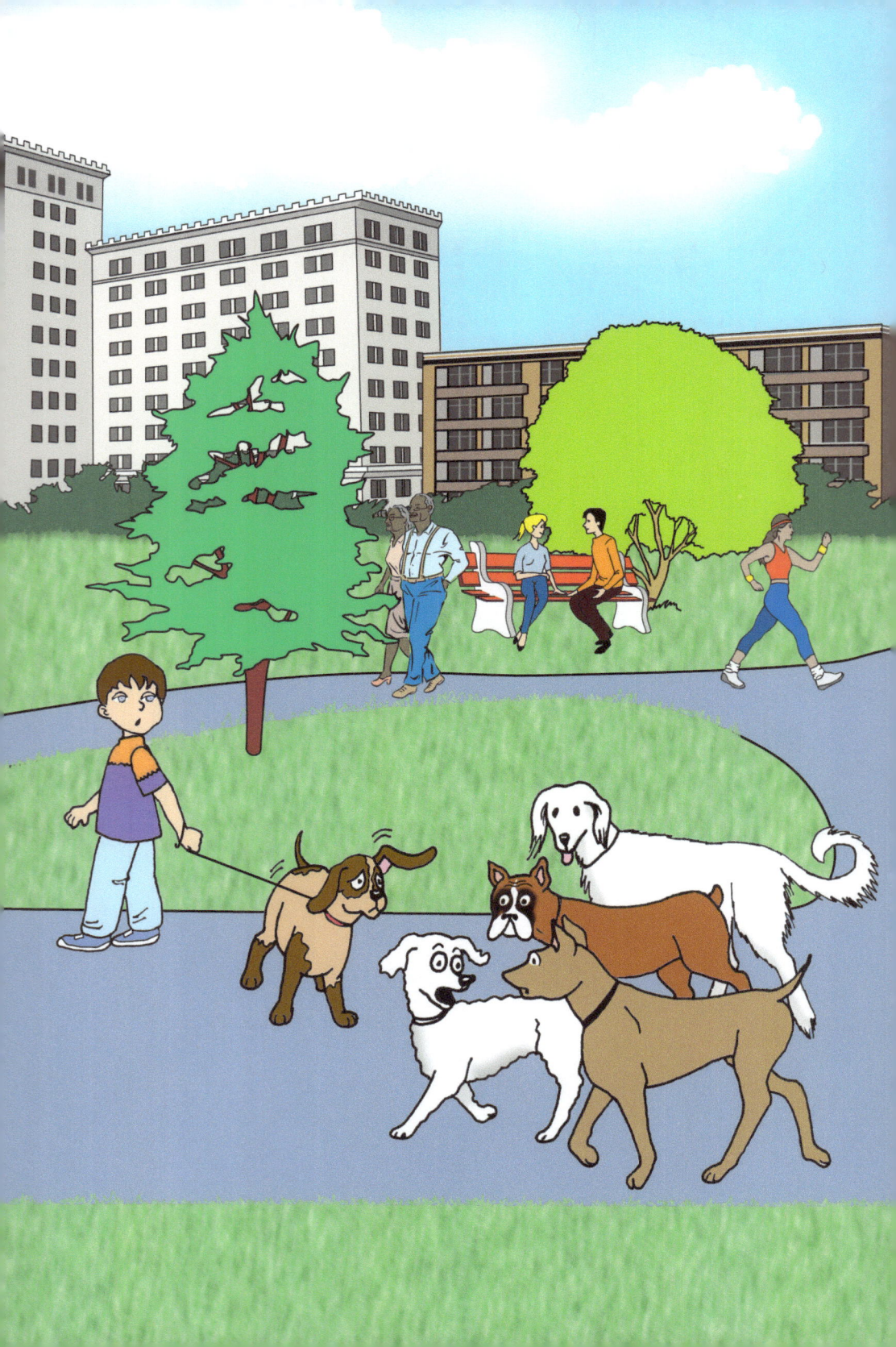

Justin's doggy, Palmer,

Went out for his walk.

With his long floppy ears,

He heard the others talk.

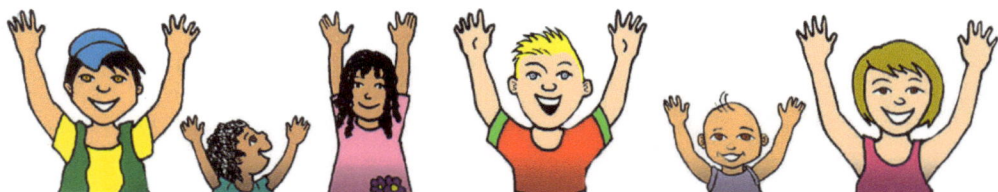

"Did you hear about Palmer's boy?"

The dogs they did not know.

"He goes to his doctor,

And he LIKES to go."

The neighbors came to visit,

To eat, to laugh, to talk.

The children went outside to play,

The grown-ups took a walk.

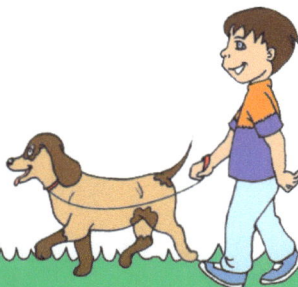

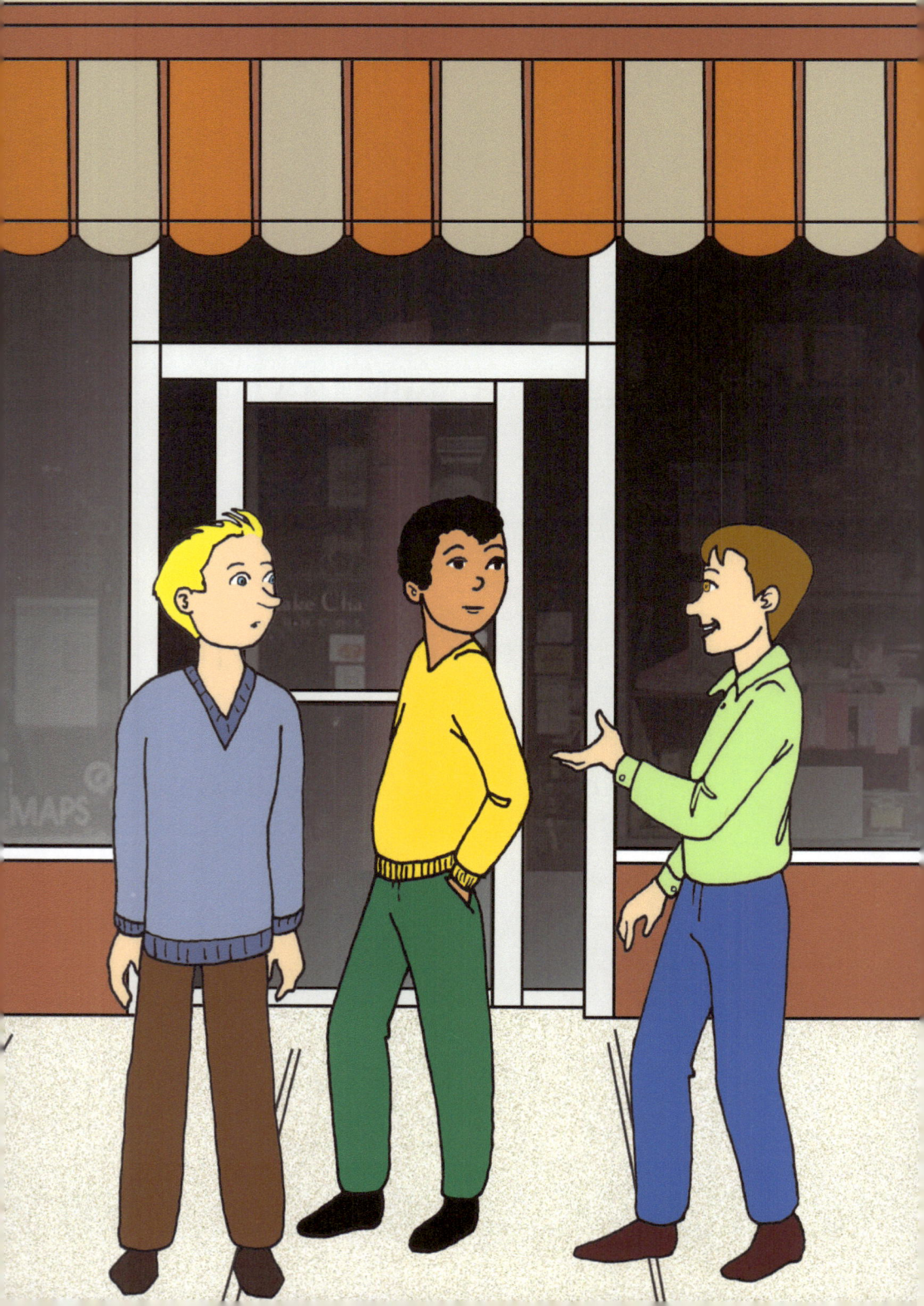

Timmy's father was confused,

"There's something I must know.

When Justin has his doctor's visit,

Does he LIKE to go?"

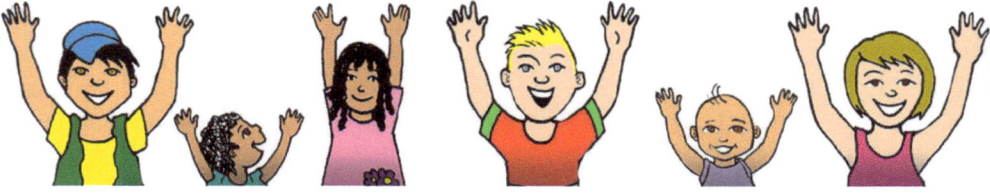

"It's true," his father said,

"One day, everyone will know.

When kids go to THIS doctor,

They really LIKE to go."

Johnny's father was surprised,

He stood with a blank stare.

"We call it an adjustment,

And it's part of wellness care."

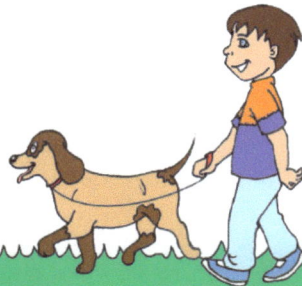

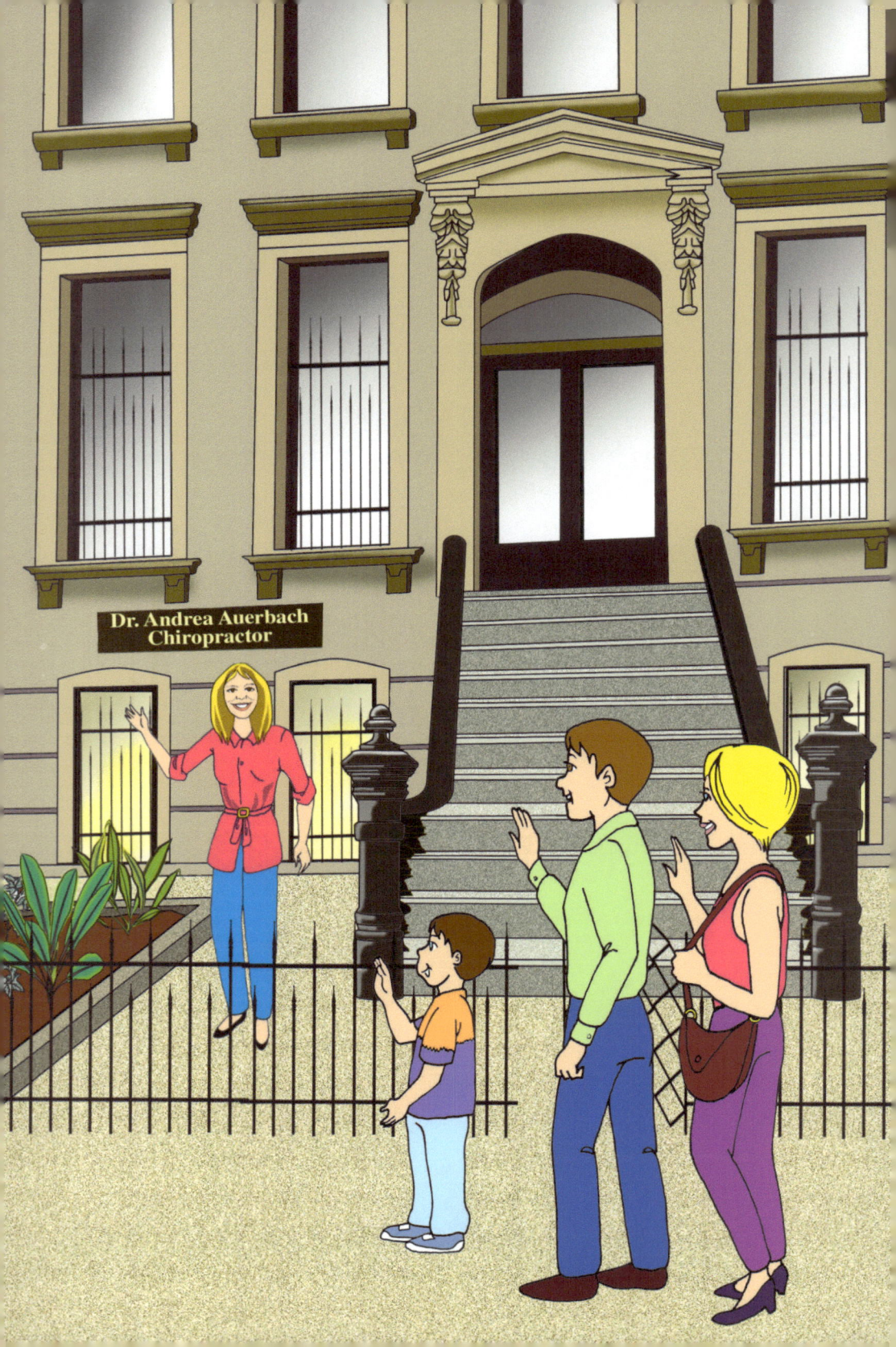

"Justin's telling you the truth,

He left out one small factor.

The doctor Justin LIKES to see,

Is Justin's CHIROPRACTOR!"

Keeping Your Children "IN TUNE"

Imagine an orchestra with multiple instruments being played in perfect harmony. If you compared the systems of the body to musicians playing various instruments in an orchestra, the nervous system would be the conductor. The conductor directs the orchestra seamlessly so that the musicians play in harmony.

Similarly, the pediatric chiropractor assumes the responsibility of keeping the child's body systems in perfect health. Beginning with the birth process, a traumatic event even under normal circumstances, a child's nervous system experiences stress from day one. The often-added obstetric interventions may cause undue force to the baby's head and neck. These stressors can cause undetected biomechanical injuries or misalignments in the spine, cranial bones, or extremities. The chiropractic term for this is subluxation.

Our perfectly designed human body protects the central nervous system with cranial and spinal bones. The brain sends messages through the spinal cord and nerves to every muscle, organ, and tissue, telling each cell how to function. Subluxations interfere with this perfect communication. Correcting them early on ensures continued nervous system health. This process is called an adjustment. Since the nervous system controls all other systems in the body, the child's immune system will also benefit.

As children develop, simple life events can cause moments of physical trauma in their bodies. Participating in sports, riding scooters and skateboards, carrying heavy backpacks, spending long hours on a computer, and simple childhood play can unknowingly stress the nervous system. Additionally, emotional challenges, environmental toxins, and improper dietary choices further stress the body. Stress leads to obstruction in the nervous system. Chiropractors are trained to evaluate and correct obstructions in the cranial and spinal structures of the body so that the body can take over and heal itself.

Chiropractic care offers an effective, conservative intervention for acute and chronic health conditions that arise in children. Infant conditions such as colic, constipation, sleep disturbances, breathing concerns, breastfeeding difficulties, digestive issues, and torticollis (head tilts) are just a few concerns that can improve with chiropractic care. Infants with no language to describe what they are experiencing find comfort in the gentle touch of the chiropractor.

Other childhood conditions that benefit from chiropractic care include: asthma, allergies, anxiety, bedwetting (enuresis), headaches, congestion, ear infections, extremity issues, scoliosis, ADD/ADHD, learning disabilities, and neurosensory disorders.

Chiropractic care can enhance function and increase comfort for children with chronic or congenital disorders such as autism, cerebral palsy, juvenile diabetes, juvenile arthritis, muscular dystrophy, and others. All children deserve the opportunity to be their personal best!

We all want our children's health to be optimal. Chiropractors can help. Getting regular chiropractic care will help your children to express their full health potential now and as they grow into adults. We invite parents to learn more about chiropractic care for children at icpa4kids.com and chirocare4kids.com.

Keeping your child's nervous system in tune sets the stage for perfect harmony!

Our Parents Speak:

"We have seen such an improvement in Gigi's health since she has been under chiropractic care. She had very low energy and was low on the growth chart. She barely talked in school, and she didn't seem happy. For the last month, she is more energetic, she's happier and more playful, and she is growing! The other parents have noticed the change, and her teacher reports that now she talks too much. We are so happy!" —Yoani Roldan

"My sons (one of whom is autistic) and I have been under Dr. A's (chiropractic) care. The kids and I always look forward to our adjustments." —Jacqueline Pierre-Louis, past president of PTA

"My son and daughter were a month old when they had their first chiropractic adjustments. They sleep better and it supports their health. It's an investment for their lives. It also helped me to have a fast delivery and my husband to keep stress levels down! We are a well-adjusted family. —Melissa Bijur

"My daughter was congested for the first eight months of her life; her breathing finally cleared when she started regular visits to Dr. A. Additionally, chiropractic treatment has helped to clear illness quickly and align her jaw." —Allison Sanchez, speech therapist

"Dr. A adjusts me and our two girls, eight and ten. We originally went to her because our ten-year-old was feeling dizzy and complaining of neck pain for a couple of months. Her pediatrician said it was anxiety. After a few sessions with Dr. A, the pain and dizziness were all gone. We started bringing our eight-year-old who'd had shoulder pain. This took about four sessions and it was gone too. My kids love going." —Kim Purcell

"My son Alex and I have been going since Alex was seven years old: he is now twelve. I first brought him for ear, stomach, and focus issues, as well as alopecia. He looks forward to getting adjusted and he always feels much better. I see a big difference in my child." —Karen Rodriguez

About the Author

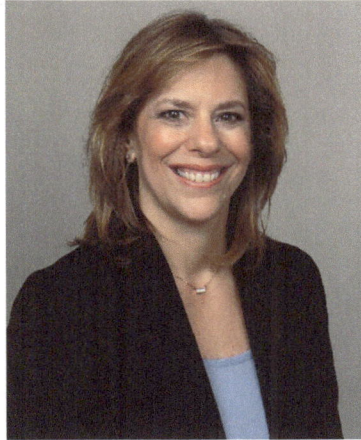

Dr. Auerbach's healing hands, warm heart, and deep concern for her patients, have made her a sought after chiropractor in Park Slope Brooklyn and its surrounding communities for over 15 years. She holds an advanced certification in pediatric and prenatal care (CACCP) from the International Chiropractic Pediatric Association and The Academy Council on Chiropractic Pediatrics. Her practice includes newborns and children of all ages, as well as adults and moms-to-be.

Dr. Auerbach's office is located at 196 6th Avenue, Brooklyn, NY, 11217. She can be reached by phone at 718-399-1111, or by email at drandreaauerbach@gmail.com. For more information about her practice, visit chirocare4kids.com.